OSTEOPOROSIS

THINGS YOU SHOULD KNOW
(QUESTIONS AND ANSWERS)

By Rumi Michael Leigh

Introduction

I would like to thank and congratulate you for purchasing this book, " *Osteoporosis, things you should know (questions and answers)*" series.

This book will help you understand, revise and have a good general knowledge and keywords of Osteoporosis and how it affects the lives of people who suffer from this disease.

Thanks again for purchasing this book, I hope you enjoy it!

Chapter 1

1) What does "osteo" signify ?

- Osteo signifies bone.

2) What does "porosis" signify ?

- Porosis signifies pore.

3) What is osteoporosis ?

- Osteoporosis is a disease that causes decrease in bone density.

4) Are bones living tissues ?

- Yes, bones are living tissues.

5) What is the name of the inner bone ?

- The name of the inner bone is the spongy bone.

6) What is the outer shell of the bone ?

- The outer shell of the bone is the compact bone.

7) What are the different types of bones ?

- The different types of bones are long, short, flat and irregular.

8) Is osteoporosis a disease ?

- Yes, osteoporosis is a disease.

9) Is bone loss a disease ?

- No, bone loss is not a disease. Bone loss is normal with aging.

Chapter 2

1) How does aging cause bone loss ?

- When we age, there is more break down of bone tissues than the creation of new ones.

2) Is genetics a risk factor for osteoporosis ?

- Yes, genetics could be a risk for osteoporosis.

3) Is osteoporosis painful ?

- No, osteoporosis is not painful.

4) Why is osteoporosis often called a silent disease?

- Osteoporosis is often called a silent disease because one can lose bone density over a long period of time without even noticing.

5) At what age do we have the peak bone mass ?

- We have our peak bone mass around age 30.

6) Does the peak bone mass happen earlier in males or in females ?

- Peak bone mass happens earlier in females than in males.

7) Can children have osteoporosis ?

- Yes, children can also have osteoporosis.

8) What are the types of osteoporosis in children ?

- The types of osteoporosis in children are idiopathic and secondary osteoporosis.

9) What is the most common type of osteoporosis in children ?

- Secondary osteoporosis is the most common type of osteoporosis in children.

10) What are the causes of secondary osteoporosis in children ?

- The causes of secondary osteoporosis in children are diabetes, leukemia, anorexia nervosa, hyperthyroidism, osteogenesis imperfecta, kidney disease, etc.

Chapter 3

1) What are the functions of the skeleton ?

- The functions of the skeleton are support, movements, protection, storage, and the formation of blood cells.

2) What is the protection function of the bone ?

- The protection function of the bone is the protection of internal organs.

3) Give some examples of organs protected by the bone.

- Some organs protected by the bone are the brain, the heart, etc.

4) What substances are stored by the bones ?

- Substances stored by the bones are mineral salts, lipids, etc.

Chapter 4

1) What are osteoclasts ?

- Osteoclasts are cells that break down old bone tissues.

2) What are osteoblasts ?

- Osteoblasts are cells that replace old bone tissues with new ones.

3) How do osteoblasts make new bone tissues ?

- Osteoblasts make new bone tissues by using minerals (phosphate and calcium) from the blood.

4) What is a secondary osteoporosis ?

- A secondary osteoporosis is osteoporosis caused by another health condition.

5) What is an idiopathic osteoporosis ?

- An idiopathic osteoporosis is osteoporosis without a known cause.

6) What race of people are susceptible to have osteoporosis ?

- White (Caucasian) and Asian people are more susceptible to have osteoporosis.

7) Why are White (Caucasian) and Asian people more susceptible to have osteoporosis ?

- White (Caucasian) and Asian people are more susceptible to have osteoporosis because they have lower levels of estrogen and testosterone levels.

8) What are some of the preventions of osteoporosis ?

- Some of the preventions of osteoporosis are :

- having a healthy diet,
- medications and
- regular physical exercise.

9) What are the risk factors for osteoporosis ?

- The risk factors for osteoporosis are :
- age
- family history,
- sex (female),
- race,
- hormones,
- tobacco,
- excessive alcohol consumption,
- lack of physical exercise,
- prostate cancer,
- breast cancer,
- kidney disease,
- lupus,
- liver disease,
- lack of sufficient calcium diet,
- etc.

10) What are the signs of osteoporosis on the vertebrae ?

- Osteoporosis can reduce a person's height and can cause the spine to curve.

Chapter 5

1) How does prostate cancer treatment increase the chances of osteoporosis in men ?

- Prostate cancer treatment increases the chances of osteoporosis in men because the treatment decreases testosterone levels.

2) How does breast cancer treatment increase the chances of osteoporosis in women ?

- Breast cancer treatment increases the chances of osteoporosis in women because the treatment reduces estrogen levels.

3) Can excessive exercises in women lead to not having menstruations ?

- Yes, excessive exercises in women may lead to not having menstruations.

4) How can tobacco cause osteoporosis ?

- Tobacco reduces the level of estrogen.

5) What is the normal value of calcium in the blood?

- The normal value of calcium in the blood is 2.25 to 2.75 mmol/L.

6) Does calcium blood test detect osteoporosis ?

- No, calcium blood test is not enough to determine osteoporosis.

7) What kind of food contains calcium ?

- The kind of food that contains calcium are dairy products such as milk, yogurt, cheese, broccoli, green vegetables, etc.

8) Why are salty foods a high risk for osteoporosis ?

- Salty foods are a high risk for osteoporosis because high levels of sodium cause calcium loss which then causes the bones to lose calcium.

9) Is caffeine consumption a risk for osteoporosis ?

- Yes, a high daily caffeine consumption is a risk for osteoporosis.

10) Why is a high daily caffeine consumption a risk for osteoporosis ?

- A high daily caffeine consumption is a risk for osteoporosis because caffeine decreases calcium absorption.

Chapter 6

1) How are osteocytes formed ?

- Osteocytes are osteoblasts that have become latent.

2) What are latent cells ?

- Latent cells are cells that are inactive.

3) What are the largest bone cells ?

- Osteoclasts are the largest bone cells.

4) Are osteoplasts really bone cells ?

- No osteoplasts are not really bone cells.

5) Is osteoporosis usually more common in men or in women ?

- Osteoporosis is usually more common in women.

6) Why do women have a higher risk of developing osteoporosis than men ?

- Women have a higher risk of developing osteoporosis than men because after menopause there is decrease in estrogen production.

7) What is usually the first physical sign of osteoporosis ?

-   A fracture is usually the first physical sign of osteoporosis.

8) What are the most common fractures associated with osteoporosis ?

-   The most common fractures associated with osteoporosis are broken wrists, broken vertebrae, broken ribs, and broken hips.

9) In patients that have risk of osteoporosis, why is there likely to be a fracture in the vertebrae, ribs, etc ?

-   There is likely to be a fracture in these areas because these bones contain mainly spongy bones.

10) Compare the spongy bone of a normal bone to the spongy bone with osteoporosis.

-   The spongy bone of a bone with osteoporosis has more pores than a spongy bone of a normal bone.

Chapter 7

1) When should osteoporosis prevention start ?

- Osteoporosis prevention should start at a young age.

2) Why should osteoporosis prevention start at a young age ?

- Osteoporosis prevention should start at a young age in order to build up enough bone mass and reduce bone loss.

3) The prevention of osteoporosis is mostly beneficial to what population ?

- The prevention of osteoporosis is mostly beneficial to the elderly, to women in the menopause phase and to prevent fractures.

4) What part of the bone does post-menopausal osteoporosis affect ?

- Post-menopausal osteoporosis affects the trabecular bone.

5) What part of the bone does senile osteoporosis affect ?

- Senile osteoporosis affects the trabecular bone and the cortical bone.

6) What is amenorrhea ?

- Amenorrhea is a lack of menstrual cycle in a woman who is still capable of having children.

7) Is amenorrhea a risk factor for osteoporosis ?

- Yes, amenorrhea is a risk factor for osteoporosis.

8) What is nulliparity ?

- Nulliparity is a woman who has never had children.

9) Is nulliparity a risk factor for osteoporosis ?

- Yes, nulliparity is a risk factor for osteoporosis.

Chapter 8

1) What kind of medications aid the bones ?

- Multivitamins and supplements aid the bones.

2) What vitamin is very important in the absorption of calcium ?

- Vitamin D is very important in the absorption of calcium.

3) What are the sources of vitamin D ?

- Some sources of vitamin D are in food intake, sunlight, and medications.

4) What are some of the medications used to treat osteoporosis ?

- Some of the medications used to treat osteoporosis are bisphosphonates, calcitonin, denosumab, selective estrogen receptor modulators (SERMS), etc.

5) What cells do medications used to treat osteoporosis act on ?

- Medications used to treat osteoporosis such as Bisphosphonates, Calcitonin, etc. act on osteoclasts.

6) What are some medications that could cause osteoporosis ?

- Medications that could cause osteoporosis include glucocorticoids, coumadin, antiseizure medications, etc.

7) What is Coumadin used for ?

- Coumadin is used for blood thinning.

8) Can medications used to treat arthritis cause osteoporosis ?

- Yes, medications used to treat arthritis can cause osteoporosis.

9) Can medications used to treat asthma cause osteoporosis ?

- Yes, medications used to treat asthma can cause osteoporosis.

Chapter 9

1) How does calcium help the heart ?

- Calcium helps in the contraction of the heart.

2) Does calcium help during blood coagulation ?

- Yes, calcium plays a role during blood coagulation.

3) What is hypocalcemia ?

- Hypocalcemia is a low calcium level in the blood.

4) What is the hormone that activates during hypocalcemia ?

- The hormone that activates during hypocalcemia is the parathyroid hormone (PTH).

5) What is hypercalcemia ?

- Hypercalcemia is a high calcium level in the blood.

6) What is the function of calcitonin ?

- Calcitonin regulates calcium and phosphorus levels in the blood.

7) Where is calcitonin secreted ?

- Calcitonin is secreted in the thyroid.

Chapter 10

1) What is osteopenia ?

- Osteopenia is the beginning of bone loss. It is a decrease in bone density.

2) Does osteopenia always lead to osteoporosis ?

- No, osteopenia does not always lead to osteoporosis.

3) What is osteogenesis imperfecta ?

- Osteogenesis imperfecta is a genetic bone disorder that causes bones to be fragile and break easily.

4) What is osteomalacia ?

- Osteomalacia is the decrease of bone mineralization.

5) What is phosphoremia ?

- Phosphoremia is the concentration of phosphorus in the blood.

6) What is the normal value of phosphoremia in an adult ?

- The normal value of phosphoremia in an adult is 40 mg/liter.

7) Parathormone acts on what organs ?

- Parathormone acts on the bone, intestine and kidneys.

8) What cells do parathyroid hormones act on ?

- Parathyroid hormones act on osteoblasts.

9) How does parathormone affect the kidneys ?

- Parathormone affects the kidneys by an increase in calcium re-absorption and by the activation of vitamin to calcitriol.

Chapter 11

1) What is BMI ?

- Body Mass Index.

2) Is BMI an indicative value for elderly people ?

- Yes, BMI is an indicative value for elderly people.

3) Why is BMI an indicative value for elderly people?

- BMI is an indicative value for elderly people because elderly people lose a few inches at the level of the vertebral column, thus the BMI calculation is an indicative value.

4) What is the BMI formula ?

- BMI = Weight (Kg)/Height (m2)

5) What is the osteodensitometry value that indicates osteoporosis ?

- The osteodensitometry value that is less than 2.6 indicates osteoporosis.

6) How is bone mineral density measured ?

- Bone mineral density is measured by the T-score.

7) What is the T-score ?

- The T-Score is the comparison/measurement of the bone mineral density relative to a normal bone density.

8) What is the Z-score ?

- The Z-score is the comparison/measurement of the bone mineral density relative to similar aged persons.

9) How is osteoporosis diagnosed ?

- Osteoporosis can be diagnosed with X-ray, blood tests, DXA scan and ultrasound.

10) What is the abbreviation DXA (scan) ?

- Dual energy X-ray absorptiometry scan.

11) What is the function of a DXA scan ?

- A DXA scan is a specialized X-ray exam used to measure bone mineral density.

Conclusion

Thank you again for purchasing this book. I hope it has helped you in your journey to understanding Osteoporosis and how it affects the people around you who suffer from it.

Thank you.